Still Me

BY REBECCA DuBOIS

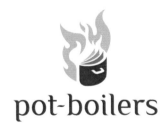

pot-boilers

Requests for permission should be made in writing to:
Pot-Boilers, 100 Stevens St. SW, Grand Rapids, MI 49507

www.stillme.com

ISBN 13 - 9780986301230

Illustrations & Book layout by
Josh Ryther & Jeremiah Elbel of Deksia

Thank you to my Heavenly Father and my family and my friends who have
provided continuous love and support to me throughout this journey.

To my friend, Ellen Van Oss,
who celebrates her cancer-free
victory in heaven.

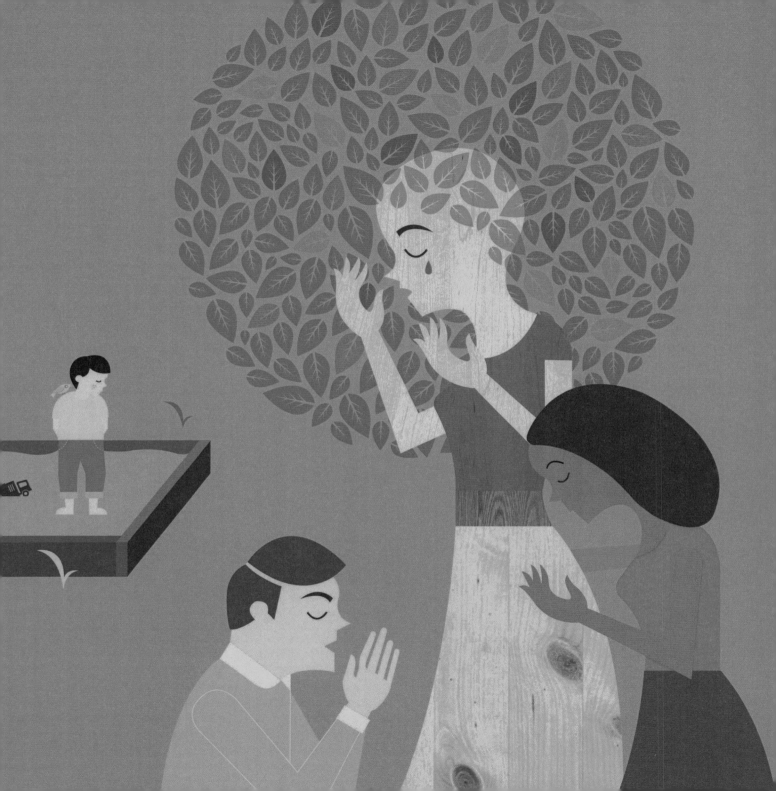

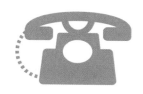

The call came on a lovely autumn day,
That changed our lives in so many ways.

"Cancer," said the doctor, "you need to prepare
For surgery, therapy, and the loss of your hair."

Mom started crying. She was very upset,
But family and friends prayed for healing instead.

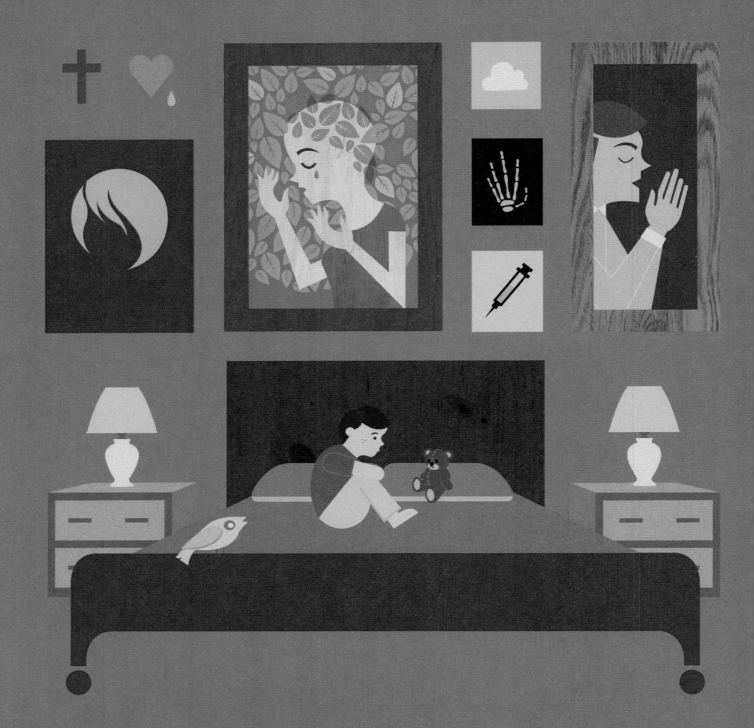

I wondered and watched in total dismay;
My world changed on that very dark day.

Questions started filling my head.
I remembered the words as I sat in my bed.

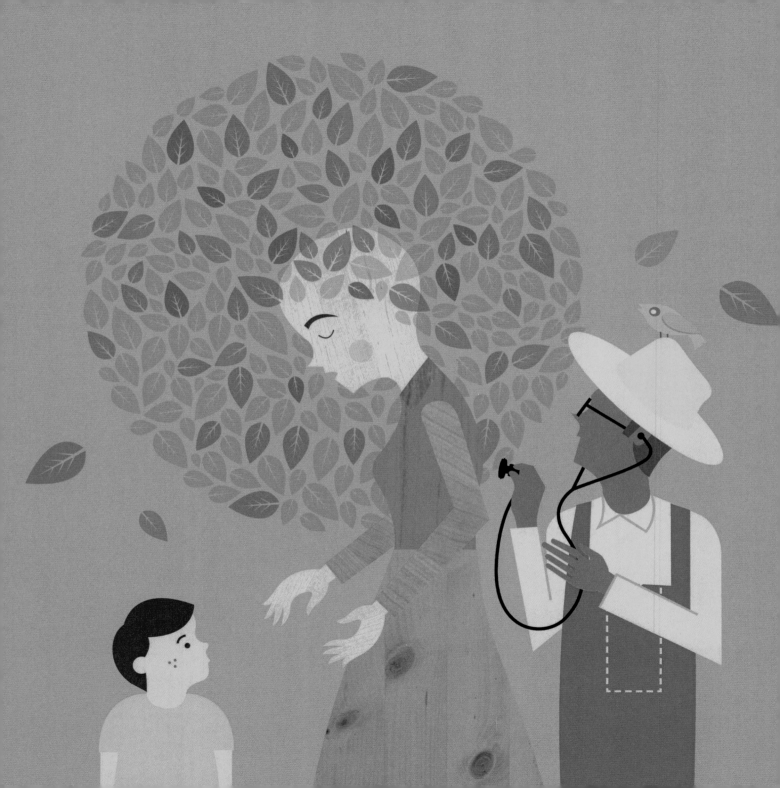

Words like fatigue, wigs, and surgery,
And what is radiation and chemotherapy?

My mind understood that cancer was bad,
And that's what made my heart so sad.

I thought of the worst, trembling with fear,
Would mom go to heaven or would she stay here?

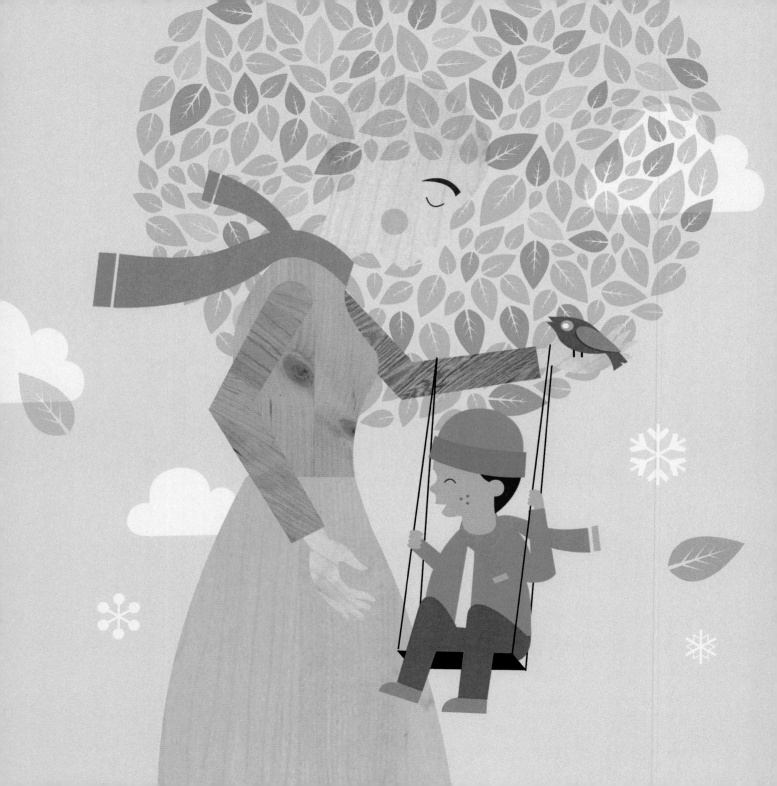

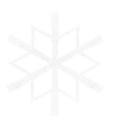

The morning brought a new attitude,
I talked with mom, and she changed my mood.

She was so strong, safe, and secure
Believing healing was coming for sure.

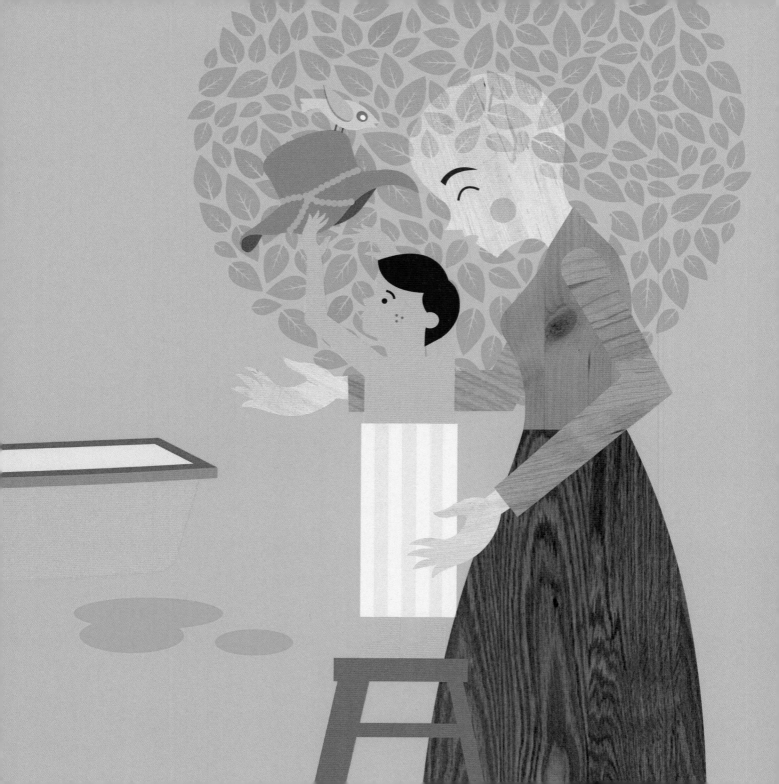

She held me tight and asked with a smile,
"Do you have fears that you've had for awhile?"

I looked in her eyes and quietly said,
"Are you going to lose all the hair on your head?"

She laughed, "Wigs and hats might change what you see,
But always remember, it's STILL ME!"

"Who will give me baths and rub my back?"
"STILL ME," she said, "I look forward to that!"

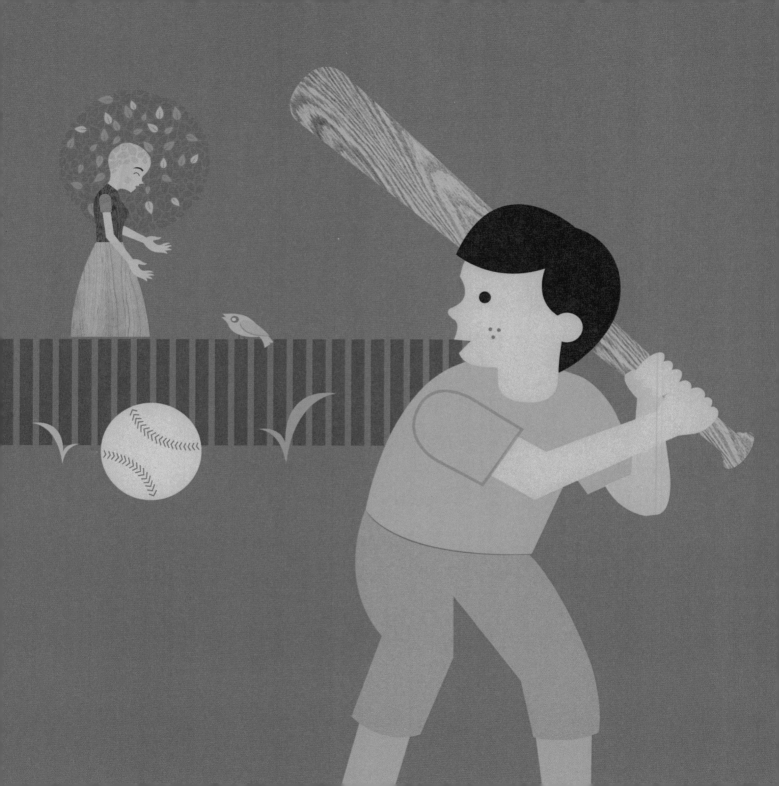

"Will you be at my baseball games?"
"STILL ME," mother said, "cheering just the same."

"And if I can't go cause I'm tired and sore,
It's STILL ME waiting for hugs at the door."

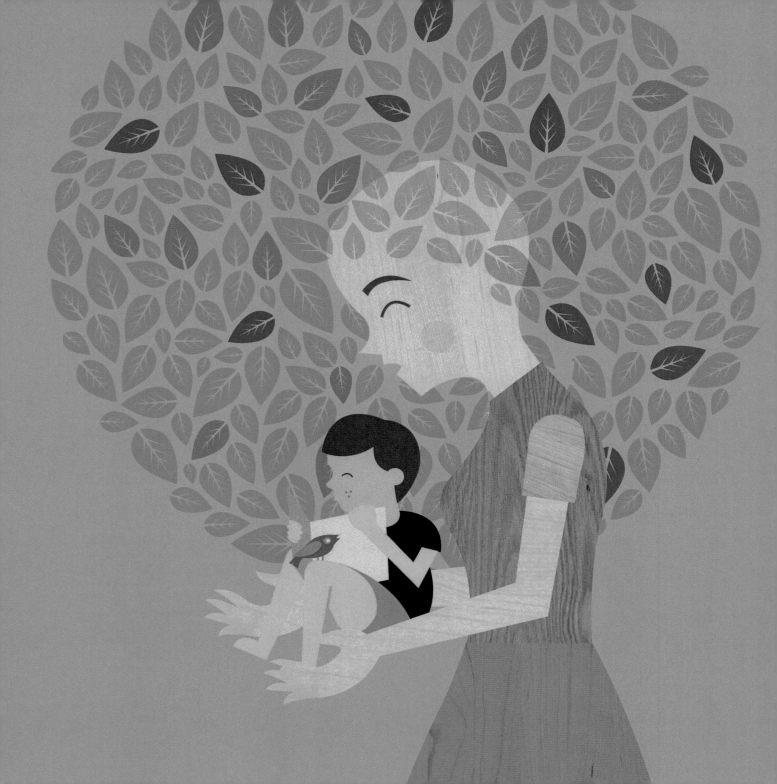

"I look forward to those times with you.
As a mother those moments will help me get through.

Like reading you books, and watching TV,
Even those times you won't listen to me."

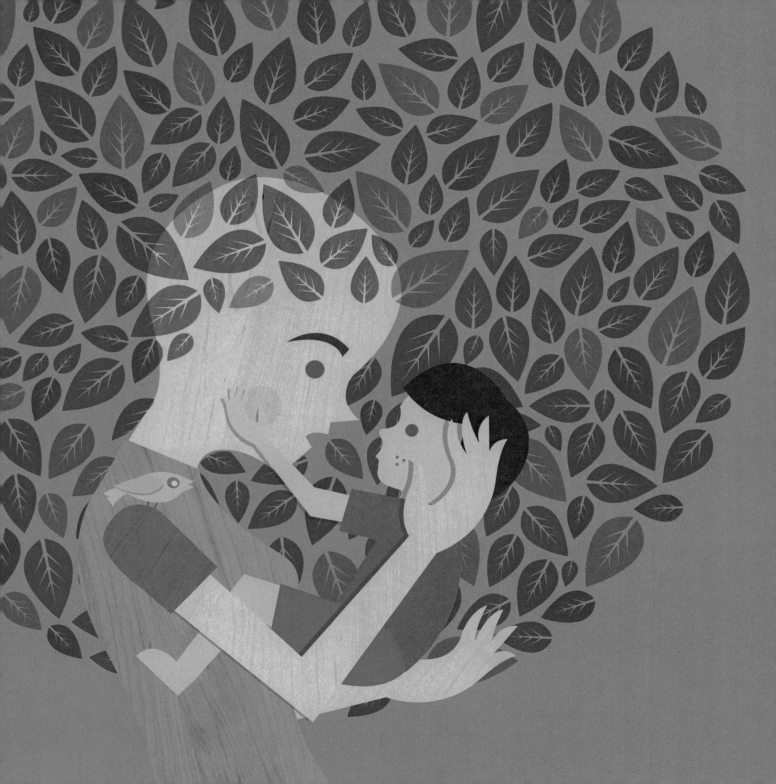

Mother looked deep into my eyes, held me close to her chest.
She uttered these words that put my fears to rest:

"God is bigger than any cancer could be.
So don't worry, God is taking care of me."

Mother has a tough battle ahead,
But with love, faith, and prayer there is nothing to dread.

When this journey is over and done,
Victory is ours. The battle is won.

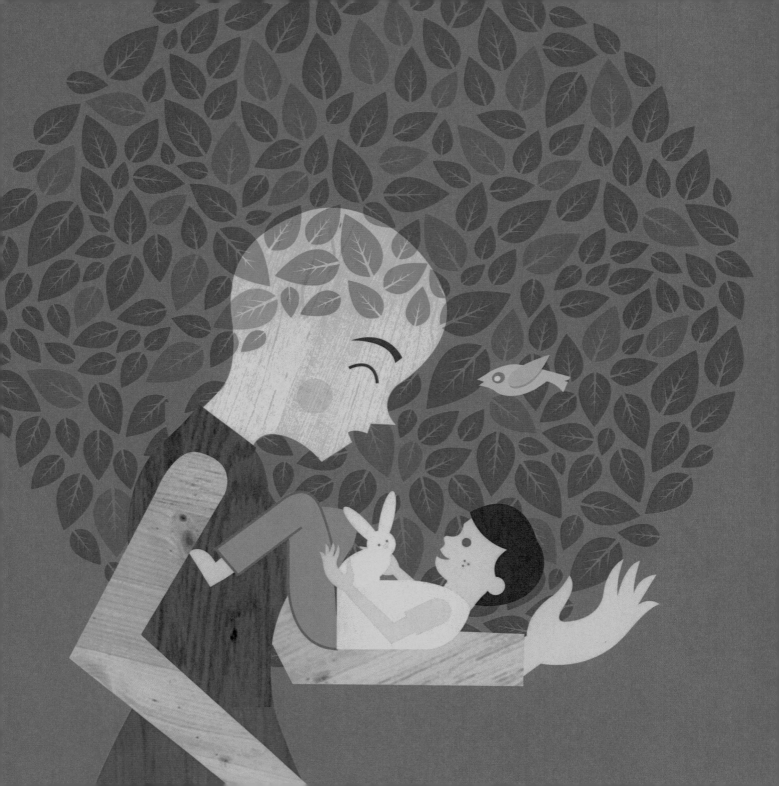

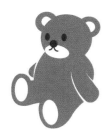

"No matter how I may look or feel,
My love for you is strong and real,

Be reassured, know, and believe
It will always and forever be STILL ME."

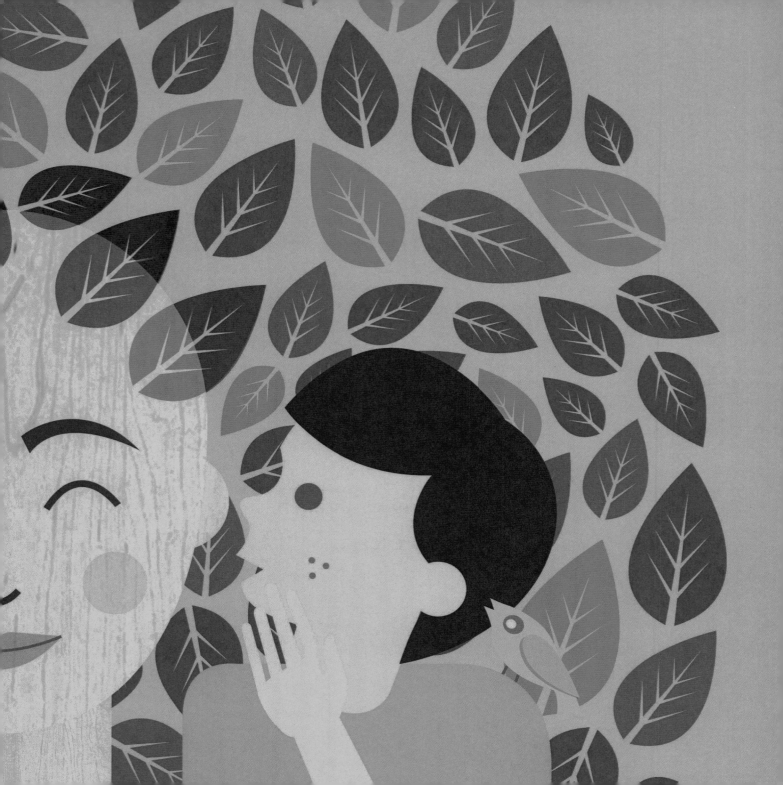

I hugged her neck tightly and said in her ear,
"It will be ME loving you, bald or with hair.
It will be ME loving you in your chemo chair.

It will be ME loving you when you're tired and sad
Or needing a pillow or having a book read."

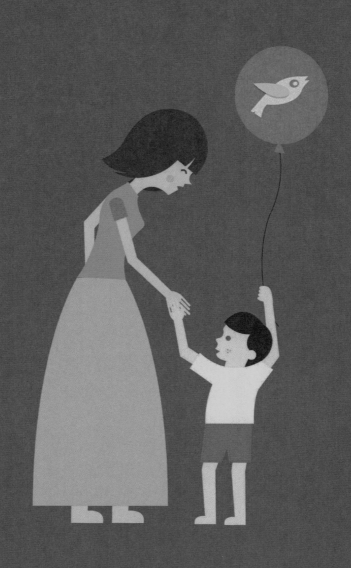

No matter what changes
may come our way,

It's STILL ME by your side,
step by step, everyday!

The End

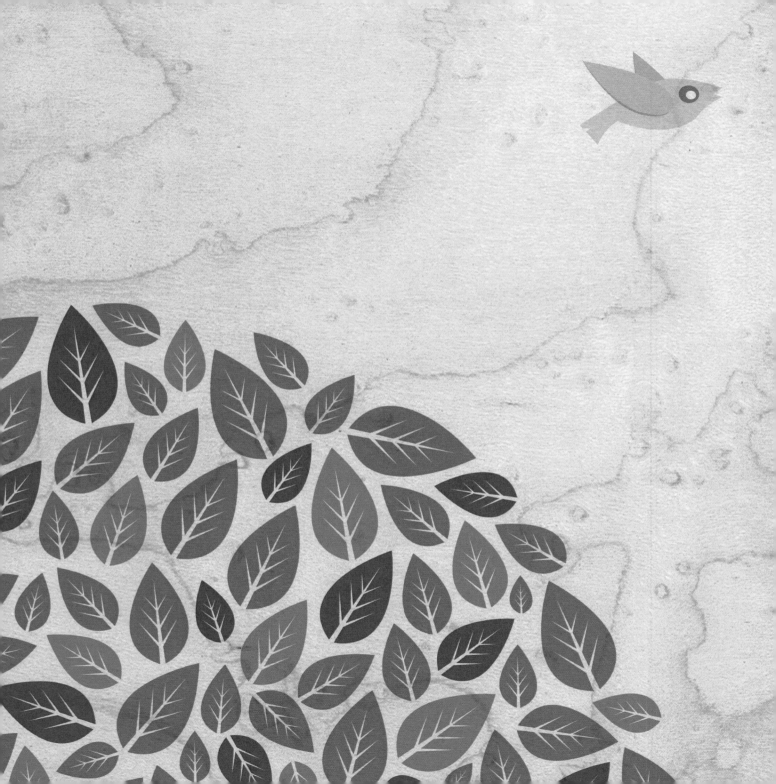